Maha Al Fahim

Curriculum, Teaching, Supervision and Assessment in Residency Training

Maha Al Fahim

Curriculum, Teaching, Supervision and Assessment in Residency Training

Scholar's Press

Impressum / Imprint

Bibliografische Information der Deutschen Nationalbibliothek: Die Deutsche Nationalbibliothek verzeichnet diese Publikation in der Deutschen Nationalbibliografie; detaillierte bibliografische Daten sind im Internet über http://dnb.d-nb.de abrufbar.

Alle in diesem Buch genannten Marken und Produktnamen unterliegen warenzeichen-, marken- oder patentrechtlichem Schutz bzw. sind Warenzeichen oder eingetragene Warenzeichen der jeweiligen Inhaber. Die Wiedergabe von Marken, Produktnamen, Gebrauchsnamen, Handelsnamen, Warenbezeichnungen u.s.w. in diesem Werk berechtigt auch ohne besondere Kennzeichnung nicht zu der Annahme, dass solche Namen im Sinne der Warenzeichen- und Markenschutzgesetzgebung als frei zu betrachten wären und daher von jedermann benutzt werden dürften.

Bibliographic information published by the Deutsche Nationalbibliothek: The Deutsche Nationalbibliothek lists this publication in the Deutsche Nationalbibliografie; detailed bibliographic data are available in the Internet at http://dnb.d-nb.de.

Any brand names and product names mentioned in this book are subject to trademark, brand or patent protection and are trademarks or registered trademarks of their respective holders. The use of brand names, product names, common names, trade names, product descriptions etc. even without a particular marking in this work is in no way to be construed to mean that such names may be regarded as unrestricted in respect of trademark and brand protection legislation and could thus be used by anyone.

Coverbild / Cover image: www.ingimage.com

Verlag / Publisher:
Scholar's Press
ist ein Imprint der / is a trademark of
OmniScriptum GmbH & Co. KG
Bahnhofstraße 28, 66111 Saarbrücken, Deutschland / Germany
Email: info@scholars-press.com

Herstellung: siehe letzte Seite /
Printed at: see last page
ISBN: 978-3-639-85947-8

Copyright © 2016 OmniScriptum GmbH & Co. KG
Alle Rechte vorbehalten. / All rights reserved. Saarbrücken 2016

Table of contents

CHAPTER 1:
THE CURRENT INTERNAL AND EXTERNAL INFLUENCES ON PLANNING AN EDUCATION PROGRAM FOR YOUR HEALTHCARE PROFESSIONAL 3
Introduction 5
Curriculum internal and external influences 6
Assessment and Evaluation 11
Conclusion 12

CHAPTER 2
THE CHALLENGES OF LARGE GROUP TEACHING AND THE PLACE OF BLENDED LEARNING IN HEALTH PROFESSIONS EDUCATION. 13
Introduction 15
Large Group Teaching 15
Making Large Group Teaching Interactive 16
Blended Learning 18
Conclusion 20

CHAPTER 3
A HANDBOOK FOR CLINICAL SUPERVISORS 21
Introduction 23
Benefits and Aims of Supervision 24
Good Supervisor Characteristics 24
Levels of Supervision 26
When to Supervise 27
On the job supervision 27
One to one meeting 30
Feedback 32
How to give feedback 32
Conclusion 34
Pocket References 35

CHAPTER 4
'ASSESSMENT FOR LEARNING AND 'ASSESSMENT OF LEARNING'
IN THE CONTEXT OF EDUCATING THE HEALTHCARE
PROFESSIONAL. 37
    Introduction..39
    Formative and Summative Assessment 39
    Assessment Methods..40
    Blueprinting 42
    Objective Structured Clinical Examination 42
    Multiple Choice Questions 43
    Portfolios for Assessment 44
    Peer Assessment..45
    Feedback 46
    Conclusion 47
    REFERENCES 49

Chapter 1:
The current internal and external influences on planning an education program for your healthcare profession.

Introduction

This chapter aims to critically discuss the internal and external influences on planning an education program for health professions. In doing so, the constraints will be evaluated while as identifying the learning opportunities and resources which can be implemented. Assessment and evaluation will also be discussed including how they are considered at the planning phase of the of curriculum development.

In planning an education program first the word "curriculum" must be clearly understood. It is derived from the latin currere which means track or race course (Prideau, 2003). Therefore this implies that the curriculum is an ongoing process rather than description of content. The curriculum has at least four elements:
1. What to teach (content)
2. How to teach (teaching and learning strategies/ instructional design)
3. Assessment
4. Evaluation

Organizing these elements into a logical pattern is called curriculum design. These elements are not separate steps but are all linked. In order to define the contents of the curriculum, the philosophy and aim should first be stated then the external and internal factors be considered in formulating its content. These factors have a direct impact on learning, although they are not part of the official or formal curriculum. The influencing factors are part of the hidden or unofficial curriculum that are part of the process of learning and are as important as the product.

Identifying these influences is important, as they may affect the planning and delivery of a program and this will therefore impact its outcomes. Addressing them will create awareness and therefore encourage more timely and informed decisions. It may also help the administrators to recognize the importance of their contribution and help guide institutions through the process, especially since some factors may be beyond their control but must still be accommodated.

Biggs' 3P (presage-process-product) model will be used to provide a structured look at the external and internal factors that are involved in curriculum planning.

Curriculum internal and external influences

Presage factors are the environmental influences in which the learning experience is carried out. These influences as mentioned earlier influence the planning, structure and outcome of the curriculum.

Developing a curriculum is a process, it reflects its assurance of quality and its recognition of all the stakeholders. In most countries, there is some form of regulation in relation to the curricula at all its stages. Some countries have set standards on how the curriculum is to be written and implemented and this therefore achieves the societal need and trend towards increased accountability. In the United Kingdom these standards are set by the General Medical Council who have also created Tomorrows Doctors document, which forms the basis of quality inspections for medical schools. While in some countries the curriculum is set by the state, in others, professional or regulatory bodies set them. In the United States the Liaison Committee on Medical Education sets the accreditation standards. In their case, as their graduates require licensure from the Liaison Committee on Medical Education, their standards must be met and therefore taken into account when developing the curriculum.

As the United Arab Emirates is a growing Country, it borrowed heavily from other countries' higher education systems, but it also created its own structure and values to meet the needs of its people. The Ministry of Higher Education and Research created standards for licensure and accreditation. With increasing globalization, especially with United Arab Emirates sizeable expatriate community, students need to be confident and assured of their qualifications. Students need to know that their qualifications are of high standards and that they will be both recognized and respected across borders, so that they have mobility between institutions and countries. Therefore in developing a new curriculum within the United Arab Emirates, standards of the licensure and accreditation will demonstrate that the curriculum is of sound international standing and that the necessary resources are being provided. Also the Ministry states that "Any institution located in the United Arab Emirates that provides regular, theoretical, practical, or applied curricula of one academic year or longer beyond the United Arab Emirates Secondary School Certification (or equivalent), and that lead to an academic degree, certificate, or diploma, must be licensed and have its programs accredited in order to be officially recognized by the Ministry". Therefore if the curriculum being developed meets this criterion, it will be imperative to meet the standards in the design of the curriculum.

To be able to compare qualifications nationally and internationally the United Arab Emirates National Framework Authority has developed a Qualifications Framework (QF). This Framework defines a set of program learning outcomes required for new qualifications at each award level. As the Qualifications Framework offers a method of national and international benchmarking for qualified individuals in the United Arab Emirates, its design ensured that it could be clearly and easily aligned to international frameworks in particular the European Qualifications Framework (EQF) and the Framework for Qualifications of the European Higher Education Area (the 'Bologna' framework). Therefore the Qualifications Framework for the United Arab Emirates comprised ten levels where, for each, learning outcome descriptions of knowledge, skills, and competence have been developed to describe the broad learning outcomes required for awarding a qualification at that level. This makes it a key question in developing a curriculum as to which level the program is to be set.

In the Arab countries including the United Arab Emirates, the Arab Board of Medical Specialties serves as the certifying body for residency training programs. They set the standards for training and develop the certifying Arab Board Examinations. Their standards are therefore a minimum requirement that must be incorporated into the curriculum.

Politics is another external influence on education and curriculum development. National philosophy and beliefs are a huge influence on education as funding may be influenced by politics. Politics may also play a role in the defining of goals, content, learning experience and evaluation strategies of the program and in hiring new personnel.

As healthcare needs vary worldwide, the medical curriculum needs to be tailored according to the countrys' or institutions' needs. Market needs can therefore be considered as an external influence on curriculum planning as it directly influences the curriculum.

The curriculum must adapt to the changing social needs. These changing needs may be national or cultural and therefore they are continuously evolving. Social influences may include religion, family structure, technology and television. For example, including the subject of sexual health in the curriculum may be an unacceptable topic in some cultures, as abortion may be an unacceptable subject in some religions. As society has its own expectations and perceptions of the profession, which is further promoted by the press and media, these factors need to be taken into account when planning and developing a curriculum.

Technology and environmental factors now have a role in the curriculum. With increased environmental awareness, depletion of resources and pollution, there is more focus on preserving resources. This may influence the curriculum by using less natural resources and relying on technology such as the Internet and computers. As technology progresses it will have a huge influence on the curriculum, students will become more independent learners with the vast amount of resources available to them through technology. It will change all aspects of the curriculum, from how and what is taught to assessment and evaluation. It will allow more flexibility in delivery in terms of location and time. Flynn and Vredevoogd (2010) state "There will be no activity in higher education that will not be affected by advances in technology".

Teachers, technical and administrative staff may be considered as internal influences that are part of presage in Bigg's 3P model. There needs to be sufficient staff to be able to deliver and support the program being developed. The staff needs to be appropriately skilled, knowledgeable and qualified. They need to be aware of both their own curriculum and the curriculum as a whole so they can put in context the learner's experience.

Teaching rooms, office space, skills labs and study rooms form part of the infrastructure. These aspects are critical in determining how the curriculum is planned, carried out and whether it will be effectively implemented and continued. Provisions have to be provided for learners at all stages of the program. There should be adequate space for both teachers and students to prepare and conduct the learning activities.

The current trends in medical education may be considered as an external influence. The trends need to be studied and addressed as they may influence the program philosophy. Recent trends in medical education show a move towards a more student-centered approach rather than the older didactic, teacher-centered approach.

One of the current trends in medical education is the move towards outcome based education and learning outcomes as a driver in curriculum planning (Harden, 2007). Outcome based education focuses away from the process model where the teaching method mattered most to a product model where learning outcomes is what matters most. Learning outcomes have replaced the time consuming and difficult instructional objectives, which had the disadvantage of being threatening to the teacher and student and ignored the complex medical practice. Its other drawback is that students found it harder to identify with these instructional objectives, as they were not learner centered. Benjamin Bloom created a taxonomy to facilitate writing learning outcomes. He created a hierarchy of complex processes in the cognitive, affective and psychomotor domains to provide a structure for writing learning outcomes. Learning outcomes show students what is expected from them in terms of knowledge, skills and attitude after finishing the program. These outcomes can therefore be used during curriculum planning and can subsequently be used in the assessment. Learning outcomes also have the advantage of engaging both teachers and students as well as giving students ownership for their own learning.

Further trends in medical education can be seen in Harden's (1984) "SPICES" model. This model shows a shift from Flexner's (1911) teacher-centered, knowledge-giving approach, to a student-centered, problem-based, integrated approach. In a student-centered approach there is more emphasis on independent learning where learning methods are tailored to the learners' needs. Therefore in developing the curriculum, details such as student's background, previous experience, disability, adult learning principles and learning styles need to be taken into account. Honey and Mumford describe four learning styles derived from Kolb's theory, activist, pragmatist, theorist and reflector. This gives an example of how adult learners may vary in the way they prefer to be taught and learn. Therefore the best curriculum is that which incorporates different teaching strategies that will encourage active student participation consequently facilitating the achievement of the learning outcomes.

Some of the internal influences on curriculum development include methods of teaching and learning. This is incorporated into the process part of Bigg's 3P model. Teaching and learning methods are also influenced by the current trends in medical education. With increasing student numbers and the use of multiple sites as well as independent student-centered learning, there is an increase in blended learning. This is being further facilitated by the information technology age. Another trend in curriculum development is the incorporation of transferable skills such as consultation skills, auditing, management skills, computer skills and leadership.

As mentioned educational strategies are considered an internal influence. With the recent trend towards integrated learning, curriculum planning has been modified from its more traditional approach. Curriculum integration breaks down the barriers between subjects therefore making it easier to develop knowledge that is more relevant to clinical practice. In vertical integration the boundaries between pre-clinical (basic science) and clinical courses are broken down. Therefore basic sciences are placed in the context of clinical practice making it more meaningful. Horizontal integration is when knowledge and skills are taught around subjects for example body systems. By doing so the relationship between disciplines is demonstrated and a more holistic view of patient problems is encouraged (Bradley and Mattick, 2008). Harden (1984) suggests that integrated learning encourages the development of a high level of objectives like demonstrating analytical and problem solving skills. Integration may also relieve the constraint of lack of resources on the curriculum by allowing the sharing of resources between departments, teachers and students. Although this may be looked at in reverse where separate departments and funding may be the internal constraint and barrier towards an integrated curriculum.

Problem-based learning is another trend in medical education and was included in Harden's (1984) "SPICES" model. It has been very influential in changing the medical curriculum across the world. Problem-based learning encourages the students to evaluate problems and cases, as they will do later in their clinical practice. This method has been shown to develop the learners' skills in problem-solving as well as encouraging independent learning and knowledge retention. The constraints to adapting problem-based learning into the curriculum may be the sizeable learning resources that may be needed. As problem-based learning requires good teamwork it may not be suitable for students with certain learning styles. For example reflectors may be intimidated and shy away from participation within the group.

Competency-based curriculum is another approach to teaching. It may be considered an internal influence as it is a method within the curriculum but it may also be influenced by accreditors such as the Accreditation Council for Graduate Medical Education who requires the curriculum to be competency-based. A competency-based curriculum is one where intended outcomes are clearly defined in terms of competencies. It requires students to complete tasks to a level of competency. These competencies can be skills, knowledge or attitudes that can be more complex as the student progresses from one year to another. The assessment strategies will then be based on the competencies so therefore need to be taken into account in the development of the curriculum.

Bligh, Prideaux and Parsell, (2001) also discussed how medical education has moved from a more teacher centered didactic approach to a student centered community based approach and the importance of taking into account these new trends in curriculum design. They discussed the "PRISMS" model of new trends, which includes practice based learning linked with professional development. This approach to teaching is more product focused and influences the curriculum by making it emphasize more on clinical practice, learning outcomes and making teaching and learning more practice based. Learning will be related to real clinical problems where students will learn by observing, practicing and discussing cases as well as receiving constructive feedback in a structured environment.

Interprofessional learning is another trend in medical education and was included in Bligh, Prideaux and Parsell, (2001) "PRISMS" model. Interprofessional learning is where students from different professional groups learn together therefore allowing them to look at a subject from different perspectives. The curriculum would have to be adapted to make the teaching more problem oriented to allow discussion, critical thinking and group work. This form of learning develops the student's skills for communication and teamwork as well as their understanding and respect for other professionals.

Assessment and Evaluation

In planning and developing a curriculum, we need to consider when a student will be ready to proceed to the next level of learning. For learning to take place there needs to be an underlying amount of baseline knowledge. The students can then build on this knowledge to understand more complex information. This is known as the spiral curriculum. Therefore in planning a curriculum, ensuring that a student can move from one stage to another can be achieved by assessment. For this reason assessment needs to be addressed in the early stages of curriculum development and can be considered as an internal influence on curriculum planning.

In designing the assessment within the curriculum, the achievement of learning outcomes should be measured. This ensures that the content has been covered. This is essential as the content, teaching and learning process and assessment need to be aligned to ensure that the intended learning outcome is achieved. This again illustrates the importance of addressing the assessment method in the planning phase of the curriculum.

A variety of assessment methods are usually needed in the curriculum to verify that the learning outcomes or competencies have been achieved. Therefore an assessment blueprint is usually used which also serves to align the teaching method with the assessment method.

Finally, in curriculum planning an evaluation process must be defined. This evaluation is intended to assemble information about the quality of the program. It identifies whether the intended outcomes and needs of the students/ stakeholders have been achieved. The evaluation also highlights successes that should be reinforced and deficiencies that need to be corrected. Dressel (1980) also discussed how the evaluation process identifies unintended outcomes of the curriculum, which then need to be addressed in the adjustment process of the curriculum.

Conclusion

Planning and developing a curriculum is a process that involves external and internal influences. Understanding these influences and their scope of involvement will help planners recognize the drivers, barriers and constraints of curriculum design and therefore help guide institutions through the process.

Chapter 2
The challenges of large group teaching and the place of blended learning in health professions education.

Introduction

This chapter critically discusses the challenges of large group teaching and the place of blended learning in health professions education. In doing so, the challenges of making large group teaching interactive will be discussed and the role of leadership in teaching and learning in higher education will also be debated.

Large Group Teaching

The lecture has been the standard method for teaching large groups and is still being used today. With globalization, increasing number of students and financial constraints it is still the most practical method of teaching for transmitting factual information to a large group of students. Some information is not available in textbooks such as new research and developments in the field; the lecture would therefore be an ideal way of transferring this information. The lecture can be a setting that can enable students to understand basic principles of a subject that can then be developed in detail by the students themselves or in study groups. Therefore till today there is a place for teaching in the large group setting despite its drawbacks.

Lectures require the student's continuous attention and concentration although Young (2009) found that there was a drop in student's attention between 10-30 minutes into the lecture, which then had a negative consequence on learning outcomes. Lecturing is a more passive activity, the students are usually busy taking notes and therefore not reflecting, formulating and asking questions. The aim of the lecture is for the teacher to be an agent that will transform knowledge to help the students interpret and construct their own knowledge and interpretation therefore the passive nature of the lecture in not conducive. Lectures are not effective in changing attitudes, they do not help the students synthesize and analyze ideas. Kolb (1984) described how learning takes place, his learning cycles describe the idea of learning as experimental i.e. learning by doing. This is particularly important in medical education as most of the learning is accomplished by doing and observing. Kolb also suggests that ideas are formed and changed through experiences and information already learned "prior learning". This therefore implies that it is essential to provide the learner with time to practice, reflect, and get constructive feedback to become an expert.

The lecturing method does not easily allow active student participation therefore providing the teacher with little feedback regarding student understanding of the delivered material. Feedback is important as it allows the teacher to assess the students' needs throughout the lecture. It can guide the teacher on how the information has been understood and what direction to focus on in future teaching activities. Students also benefit from feedback as it gives them information on their knowledge and understanding.

It is therefore important to develop ways of teaching that can both accommodate large groups and make the students more engaged in the learning process. One way of achieving this is by making large group teaching interactive.

Making Large Group Teaching Interactive

Interactive lecturing may be defined in a number of ways but most of the literature agrees that it implies the active involvement and participation by the students so that they are no longer passive in the learning process (Steinert and Snell, 1999). This therefore promotes active learning, students motivation and attention, gives the teacher and student feedback which enhances the satisfaction of the teacher and student.

There are many ways to make large group teaching more interactive. One technique is to tell the students what they are meant to learn at the start of the lecture. This can be done with an overhead slide giving subheadings to the lecture with some explanation or a diagram. By doing this students will know what learning outcomes are expected of them and will allow them to concentrate during the important parts of the lecture. Personalizing the class is another technique that can be used to make the students more comfortable. Students find large classes impersonal and are therefore less likely to engage and ask questions. By simply asking neighboring students to introduce themselves to each other or getting them to complete short biographical questionnaires with names, hobbies etc, students will feel more at ease.

Buzz groups are another method of making the lecture interactive. Students can group in two's or four's among neighbors without any moving to discuss a topic for a few minutes. This technique helps the students to correct their understanding and gives the teacher instant feedback over the class understanding. This can also be achieved by using an electronic response system. Not only does it give instant feedback but it also stimulates the audience attention. It has the advantage of being anonymous which reassures the student and promotes participation and honesty. This then allows them to compare their performance to their colleagues. The disadvantage to this method is that only closed questions can be answered.

Many students find it difficult to listen, concentrate and write notes in a lecture. While taking notes a certain amount of the ideas from the lecture may be missed. Students should be given time to reflect on the bigger picture to stimulate higher order thinking. Techniques such as distributing written material or handouts of slides may be helpful. For example, one study showed that students preferred to write in the space between headings, and the more space left, the more notes were taken (Newble and Cannon, 1994). Recording the lecture and making it available to the students in the library or on line will also help students to concentrate and reflect more in class. This technique would be especially helpful to international students whose English may not be their first language.

Bligh (1971) found that in a lecture students had an attention span of about 10 to 15 minutes. A change in activity every 15 minutes restored performance to almost the original level. Therefore a change in educational technology such as using audio, video, audiovisual aids, clinical cases and role-plays will maintain the students concentration.

Interactive lecturing is particularly important in medical education as the application and use of information is important for problem solving, communication skills and decision-making. Students are required to think more on their feet, which makes it important to apply the information rather than recall facts.

Blended Learning

Blended learning can be defined as a combination of face-to-face teaching and on-line learning. This form of teaching is being implemented worldwide to adapt to globalization, increasing number of students and inadequate infrastructure to accommodate them. Therefore, whilst discussing the methods of making large group teaching interactive, another way to deal with large group teaching is to introduce blended learning.

Blended learning encourages wider participation of students in learning. It enables access to some students who may not have been able to otherwise take part in higher education

(Macdonald and Stratta, 2001). These students include part time students who cannot attend daily classes due to other commitments, disabled students and long distance learners.

Recent themes and trends in medical education have been driving the move towards blended learning. Student centeredness is one such theme. As there are a wide variety of physical environments in which teaching and learning can occur, in clinical teaching, this may be at the patient's bedside, in an outpatient clinic, in the operating theatre, in a skills laboratory (virtual learning), lecture theatre, small group learning as well as e-learning. Clinicians and teachers therefore have been changing their approach from delivering teaching to facilitating learning. This shift from teacher centeredness to a student-centered approach is a new trend in education, which gives the student a high level of responsibility for managing their learning.

Another drive towards a blended approach to teaching and learning is the new trend and concept of 'lifelong learning'. In medicine, information and knowledge changes and develops very rapidly, making it important for students to know where to find the information they are seeking than for them to know the answer. Students will have to continue to learn and keep up with information throughout their lives; therefore they need to acquire skills such as self-motivation, study skills, and take responsibility for their own learning.

One of the less mentioned but highly important benefits of blended and online learning is the information literacy and information technology skills that it provides students, these new abilities will benefit them throughout their entire academic and employment years (Dziuban, et al., 2004). This ability would be considered a transferrable skill, which is fundamental to the principles of adult learning.

As many clinical teachers are very busy on their service, a blended learning approach may help facilitate teaching and learning, teachers may provide on-line learning materials, links to resources and establish on-line group discussion. This can prepare the students for the face-to-face interaction such as lectures, problem based learning sessions, tutorials etc. This leads to a more student-centered approach, which gives the students more responsibility for their own learning.

For institutions to introduce blended learning, the content, format, recipient and time must be considered. Curricula or courses have aims, specific learning objectives or outcomes, therefore the learning activities and modes of delivery should be designed to allow students to achieve these learning objectives. Subsequently a valid and reliable assessment needs to be designed to measure the students learning and finally an evaluation to review the new teaching methods ensuring constructive alignment.

Institutions also need to deal with the administrative, financial, academic, ethical, technological and student issues. Leaders in education need to assess the preparedness of the institution or organization, the availability of the infrastructure, learners' needs and the financial implication of blended learning. Studies have shown that there is a high cost encountered in the development of the e-learning materials (Gunasekaran, et al., 2002). However, since these materials can be reused, eventually the savings will cover the initial cost. Then, there comes the continuous cost of maintaining and updating the e-learning materials which must not be overlooked, which Heinze (2008) suggests may be covered with the fee income from increasing student numbers that blended learning brings. A needs analysis should be performed to assess the learners' needs and the requirements for a blended form of teaching and learning.

Leaders need to also take into consideration staff development, as it is essential for the implementation of blended teaching and learning. "Just as students have to relearn how to learn, faculty have to relearn how to teach" (Heinze, 2008). As not all staff engage in the process of change, and that includes new approaches in teaching and learning, leaders need to communicate the vision clearly, gain buy-in from all stakeholders then subsequently facilitate the process of change.

Conclusion

The lecture has been the standard method for teaching large groups and is till being used today. With globalization, increasing number of students and financial constraints it is still the most practical method of teaching for transmitting factual information to a large group of students. Another way to deal with large group teaching is to introduce blended learning, which encourages larger student participation, suits adult learners more by being more student centered, encourages active learning, provides transferrable skills and accommodates different learning styles.

Leaders in education need to be aware of the needs and recourses available to them, to allow them to enhance teaching and facilitate learning. They need to continuously adapt then evaluate to review the new teaching methods.

Chapter 3
A handbook for clinical supervisors

Introduction

Why a handbook for clinical supervision?
Doctors are trained to treat patients and not to supervise, although they are often expected to supervise, teach and evaluate students. They do the task with little experience and often find it challenging. Clinical supervision is vital in medical education although it is the least discussed and developed aspect of clinical teaching. As there is a limited amount of literature focusing on clinical supervision, this handbook aims to offer a practical and informative guide to good clinical supervision.

Who is it for?
This handbook is for anyone who supervises in the clinical setting particularly in resident supervision, although it may also be relevant and applicable to interns and medical students. This handbook can also be of benefit to those leading and managing the educational training.

What is Supervision?
Defining supervision may be complex as it may take a variety of names and forms. These include educational supervision, clinical supervision, learning support, coaching and mentoring. People seem to take a different approach depending on their professional agenda, background and experience. Essentially the basis and common element of these terms includes performance monitoring and standard setting (Kilminster, et al., 2002).

One broad definition by Kilminster (2007), defines supervision as the provision of guidance and feedback on matters of personal, professional and educational development in the context of trainee experience of providing safe and appropriate patient care.

Depending on the agreement between the supervisor and the trainee, supervision can focus on a clinical case, performance or development. At times the supervisor is only overseeing the trainee on a clinical case, such interactions are common on busy wards or clinics. On other occasions, supervision focuses on performance of the trainee, whether on a clinical rotation, specialty or task. To a lesser extent in clinical practice is supervision that focuses on development, which is mentoring and coaching. In most cases the 3 overlap as coaching and mentoring often occur, although they are not officially labeled.

Benefits and Aims of Supervision

Generally in healthcare, supervision, whether clinical, educational or managerial, aims at ensuring patient safety and promotes professional development through reflection.

Supervisors monitor that students meet standards and follow the rules; this therefore ensures quality and patient safety. There is also evidence that good clinical supervision improves morale and job satisfaction and may even prevent stress and burnout (Sloan, 2006). Having support from supervisors allows the students to share their anxiety, identify stressors and together formulate tools to deal with them.

From a supervisee perspective, having a supervisor may help inspire and promote performance, both clinically and professionally. The supervisor may act as a role model in the personal or professional sense, therefore developing the trainee's knowledge, confidence, self-awareness and endurance.

Finally, supervision also promotes reflective practice. By sharing knowledge and allowing the student to reflect, identify strengths and deficiencies, the supervisor may then guide and facilitate opportunities for further development.

Good Supervisor Characteristics

An effective supervisor needs to have the following characteristics and skills.
1. Clinical Competence
Supervisors need to be knowledgeable clinicians and have up to date knowledge and skills in their field in order to be credible. They need to be able to guide the students in linking theory to practice as well as to problem solve.

2. Good Interpersonal Skills
Good communication, counseling and listening skills are essential. Supervisors need to be respectful, empathetic, supportive, positive and enthusiastic.

3. Teaching Skills

Effective supervisors are those who genuinely enjoy teaching, have an interest and knowledge of teaching and learning principles. Supervisors need to know how to evaluate the student therefore need to be familiar with the learning objectives.

4. Positive Role Model

Supervisors are not only teaching the written curriculum but also the hidden curriculum, which includes professionalism. Therefore being a positive role model is an essential characteristic for supervisors.

Characteristics of a Role Model
• Capable clinician and teacher
• Knowledgeable of self limitations
• Reflective and admits mistakes
• Demonstrates good citizenship in workplace and community
• Enthusiastic about patient care and teaching
• Empathetic and respectful towards patients and learners
• Ethical, professional and dignified
• Interested in learners experience
• Develops good rapport with learners
• Accessible to learners
• Non Judgmental in critiquing learners

(Reed and Wright, 2010)

5. Gives Feedback

Giving feedback is one of the supervisors' most important roles. Students need to know about their strengths, weaknessess and how to improve; therefore giving effective feedback is crucial.

6. Attends supervisor training courses

There is evidence that training has a positive effect on supervisors. Training usually includes teaching methods, giving feedback, assessment, counseling skills and principles of supervision.

It is also important to highlight the ineffective supervisory behaviors so that they may be avoided. The research shows, mainly from student surveys, that undesirable supervisor characteristics include:
1. Being negative
2. Being rigid
3. Lacking empathy
4. Failing to teach
5. Humiliating
6. Unsupportive
7. Impatient and Intolerant

Levels of Supervision

ACGME states "residents must be supervised by teaching staff in such a way that the residents assume progressively increasing responsibility according to their level of education, ability and experience".

Therefore residents earn progressive responsibility for the care of the patients and it is the decision of the supervisor as to which activities the students will be allowed to perform within the context of the assigned levels of responsibility.

Typically the content of what is supervised at different levels will change, but the level of supervision will depend on the student and their relevant experience. The supervisors will need to make judgments as to whether they need to be:

- Present in the same room as the person being supervised, providing direct supervision (direct supervision)

- Nearby and immediately available to come to the aid of the person being supervised (immediately available supervision)

- In the hospital or primary care premises and available at short notice, able to offer immediate help by telephone and able to come to the aid of the person within a short time (local supervision)

- On call and available for advice, able to come to the trainee's assistance in an appropriate time (distant supervision).

Logbooks and portfolios can be useful tools in helping to determine the level of supervision required. (Kilminster, 2007)

When to Supervise

Supervision will vary from specialty to specialty, depending on the nature of the specialty (surgical or non surgical) and the location, for example hospital or primary healthcare center. The common element is that students will be supervised with regards to their knowledge, attitude and skills as they progress in their training ensuring patient safety, trainee safety and quality of service.

Students primarily need to be supervised in two separate settings. The first being 'on the job' supervision the second is one to one scheduled meetings.

On the job supervision

This usually occurs on the wards or clinics and usually focuses on clinical cases. As the clinical supervisor commonly faces the challenge of delivering quality patient care and still have the time to teach effectively, tools like the one-minute preceptor help make such tasks simpler. This technique was first described in 1992 and is still being used today. The one-minute preceptor allows both the learner and teacher to identify knowledge gaps and therefore focus learning (Neher et al., 2003).

The one-minute preceptor technique is suited for both the inpatient and outpatient setting as most of the clinical teaching involves the students interviewing then examining the patients followed by presenting the case to the supervisor.

How Time is Spent Teaching

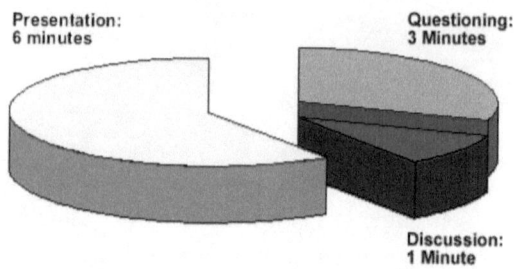

med-ed.virginia.edu

As shown above, the teacher and supervisor encounters usually takes about ten minutes with most of the time being spent on the case presentation, this will therefore leave only one minute for the discussion. Using the steps of the one-minute preceptor allows the supervisors to use the full encounter to maximize the teaching.

The One-Minute Preceptor Steps

The One-Minute Preceptor consists of a number of steps that are used at the end of the case presentation.

One Minute Preceptor Steps
1. Get a commitment
2. Probe for supporting evidence
3. Teach a general rule
4. Reinforce what was done well
5. Correct mistakes and discuss next steps

Step One: Get a Commitment

The first step is used immediately after the student presents a case. The objective is to get the student to process the information just collected from the patient by getting them to verbally commit to an aspect of the case. This can be done by asking questions such as: "What do you think is going on?" or "What do you want to do?" Doing so allows the supervisor to obtain information on the student's clinical reasoning ability and also gives a sense of involvement and responsibility in the patient care.

Step Two: Probe for Supporting Evidence

Once the student has made a commitment, the supervisor needs to explore the basis of the decision. The student's basic knowledge and ability to connect different pieces together is important to rule out the lucky guesses. Therefore questions such as "What led you to that conclusion?" and "What else did you consider?" will demonstrate the use of appropriate supporting evidence.

Step Three: Teach A General Rule

The goal at this step is to target teaching properly. By identifying the student's knowledge gaps, the supervisor is then able to teach one or more general rules that are related to the case. Supervisors need to avoid the common mistake of trying to teach too much on a single case. As the students can only integrate a few general rules per case, supervisors will have to focus on the most important areas.

Step Four: Reinforce What Was Done Well

Students need to know what they did well to improve. Supervisors' comments need to be specific in terms of knowledge, skills or behaviors that are being reinforced. Doing so increases the likelihood that the students will replicate these positive skills and attitudes into the next patient encounters.

Step Five: Correct mistakes and discuss next steps

Telling students which areas need improvement is vital for their learning. In this step, the supervisor gives specific comments that are related to performance on the case with suggestions on alternate actions or behaviors in order to direct the student in future similar cases.

Supervisors may find the five steps of the one-minute preceptor difficult to remember when first used and practiced, therefore a cut out card with the five steps has been added to the end of this handbook. The card may be cut out and carried easily in the pocket, which will help keep the steps in mind.

One to one meeting

This is usually a pre-scheduled meeting that focuses on exploring different issues. One to one meetings need to be scheduled for the following seasons.

1. Beginning of a rotation

Supervisors need to meet with their trainees at the start of each rotation. The purpose of this meeting is to discuss the goals and objectives of the rotation and how they will be taught. Students expectations should also be addressed and work schedule agreed on.

2. Mid Rotation

Supervisors need to meet with students during the mid point of the rotation to give constructive feedback on the student's performance and for any deficiencies to be identified and communicated with an agreed action plan.

3. End of Rotation

Supervisors frequently submit the end of rotation evaluations without discussing them with the students. Constructive feedback is critical for performance improvement. A meeting should to be set by the supervisor close to the time of the end of the rotation to make it more effective. How to give constructive feedback will be discussed later in the handbook.

4. Semi Annual Evaluation

This evaluation is a required by the ACGME. The program director is responsible for providing each resident with a documented semi-annual evaluation of performance with feedback.

5. Annual Evaluation and Appraisal

The annual evaluation and appraisal is a requirement of the ACGME. The supervisor, in this case the program director, needs to submit a documented evaluation, which has already been discussed and agreed on by the student.

6. Remediation

Part of the supervisors' tasks is to identify, support and guide the students in difficulty. They need to be familiar with both the human resources and education institute policies and procedures in order to comply with both. Generally about 10% of students will have some difficulty during their training (NSW IMET, 2009).

Students most commonly face problems on three issues
1. Work performance, for example poor clinical skills compared to peers,
2. Poor professional conduct and behavior, e.g. aggressive behavior
3. Physical and mental health issues, such as depression.

It is important for supervisors to be able to identify the early signs of students in difficulty. Examples of such behaviors include not answering pagers, defensiveness and excessive amount of sick leaves. The supervisor's role will include assessing the severity of the situation to identify whether patient safety or student safety have been compromised or if there is evidence of criminal conduct. After confidential discussion with the student, supervisors then need to refer the trainee to the appropriate source. In most cases this will be the program director who may then refer the case to the clinical competency committee.

Research has shown that for effective supervision to occur there has to be an active involvement of both the student and supervisor. A time needs to be set in advance of the scheduled meeting. This time needs to be protected in terms of space and time with no interruptions to allow the students to feel they are in a safe and trusting environment. This is also maintained by keeping the contents on the discussion confidential. Only if there is an issue of unsafe practice should this confidentiality be broken.

Students may have negative feelings when hearing the word supervision, therefore they need to be educated about supervision, to understand what it is and what it is not. It is important to discuss the goals and objectives that the meeting will focus on, which needs to be agreed upon by both the student and supervisor.

It is important that the supervisor role models positive behaviors during supervision by demonstrating respect, reliability, punctuality and availability. This will serve to establish a trusting relationship between the supervisor and student and most likely pass on these behaviors to the student.

A positive supervisory experience has many benefits; it can boost the student's morale and increase self-confidence. If the student feels safe and supported they will gradually take more risks with the relationship (Sloan, 2006).

Feedback

Feedback is an essential part of medical education. It allows the students to maximize their potential and draws attention to their strengths and weaknesses, allowing plans to be made to improve the deficiencies (William, et al., 2007).

Students value feedback and research suggests that students feel they are not getting enough (Gil, et al., 1984). Without feedback, mistakes can go uncorrected, and bad habits can develop, good performance is not reinforced and student may not reach their potential.

How to give feedback

Specific characteristics have been found to contribute to effective feedback in supervision. The "IMPROVE" strategy can help supervisors through the feedback process.

Give Feedback To Help Learners IMPROVE
I   Identify rotation objectives with the learner
M Make a feedback-friendly environment
P assess **Performance**; Prioritize the feedback you give
R Respond to the learner's self-assessment
O Objective: report specific behaviors observed; describe potential outcomes of behavior
V Validate what the learner has done well or suggest alternative strategies
E Establish a plan to implement changes (if needed); have learner summarize feedback and plan

I- Identify rotation objectives with the learner

This step involves preparing the student for the feedback. The goals and expectations of the student should have been discussed at the beginning of the rotation making this step easier, avoiding surprise and confusion. The student should also be told at the initial visit that feedback would be given at both the middle and end of rotation so the student will not be surprised.

M- Make a feedback friendly environment

As discussed earlier, the environment the feedback is given in is vital. This can be achieved by showing enthusiasm and interest in the learner's performance. Questions about the learners career goals and linking it to the rotation is sometimes helpful. Supervisors should verbalize that the goal is to work together towards a common goal.

P- Assess performance, P- Prioritize what feedback to give

The best method of assessing the student's knowledge, skills and attitude is through direct observation. It is also helpful to hear what other staffs have observed. Additionally the ACGME requires 360 feedback of each student making it a requirement to also have student feedback from faculty, resident peers, nurses, managers and clerks.

Too much feedback will make it difficult for the student to retain all the information. Therefore the supervisor needs to identify up to five important points.

The "sandwich" technique can also be used which starts and ends with the positive feedback, sandwiching the criticism in between. Although most students are now familiar with this technique and tend to dismiss the positive criticism feeling that the supervisor is simply trying to sugar coat the criticism.

R- Respond to learner's self assessment

Before the supervisor gives their assessment, students should be asked to reflect and make their own assumptions. Reflection on their own performance allows the student to assimilate concepts, skills, knowledge and values into their preexisting knowledge, which then promotes the intellectual growth of the student (William, et al., 2002).

O- Be Objective- Describe specific behaviors observed

The feedback given should be specific, based on direct observation of the student. These specific observations need to be described and should not be subjective.

V- Validate positive behaviors or suggest alternative strategies

This is the stage when the positive behaviors are reinforced and alternate behaviors are suggested.

E- Establish a plan

Supervisors need to make a plan or strategy to improve the student's weak performance areas, for example set reading plans.

Conclusion

When clinical supervision is carried out in a supportive and trusting manner it becomes an essential process that contributes significantly to quality patient care and safety. The quality of the supervision has been shown in the literature to be the single most important factor in determining the effectiveness of the supervision. Therefore the supervisors need to continuously self appraise and reflect on their own skills and make changes to their style if needed.

Supervision is a continuous process and does not stop after completion of training. It is part of life-long learning and helps the supervisee face new challenges through both reflection and professional conversations. This consequently contributes to job satisfaction and improved work performance.

Pocket References

Characteristics of a Role model

- Capable clinician and Teacher
- Knowledgeable of self limitations
- Reflective and admits mistakes
- Demonstrates good citizenship in medical workplace and community
- Enthusiastic about patient care and teaching
- Empathetic and respectful towards patients and learners
- Ethical, professional and dignified
- Interested in learners experience
- Develops good rapport with learners
- Accessible to learners
- Non Judgmental in critiquing learners

Give Feedback To Help Learners IMPROVE

I Identify rotation objectives with the learner
M Make a feedback-friendly environment
P assess Performance; Prioritize the feedback you give
R Respond to the learner's self-assessment
O Objective: report specific behaviors observed; describe potential outcomes of behavior
V Validate what the learner has done well or suggest alternative strategies
E Establish a plan to implement changes (if needed); have learner summarize feedback and plan

One Minute Preceptor Steps

1. Get a Commitment
2. Probe for Supporting Evidence
3. Teach a General Rule
4. Reinforce What Was Done Well
5. Correct mistakes and discuss next steps

Chapter 4
'Assessment for learning and 'assessment of learning' in the context of educating the healthcare professional.

Introduction

This chapter critically discusses 'assessment for learning and 'assessment of learning' in the context of educating the healthcare professional.

The word assessment is derived from the Latin word assidere, which means 'to sit beside'. This gives a picture of a teacher sitting besides a student helping them to learn rather than testing their performance (Swaffield, 2011). This shows that Assessment's fundamental role in medical education does not only serve for licensing, certifying and selecting students but also plays a role in motivating students to learn, hence the phrase 'assessment drives learning'. Furthermore Assessment can give teachers an indication of the effectiveness of their teaching, through their student's performance, this can also be seen as quality assurance. Areas of weakness can be identified where the course can then be reviewed and improved.

The General Medical Council in the UK has made recommendations concerning student assessment and performance. They suggest that method of assessment must support the curriculum and allow students to prove that they have achieved the curricular outcomes. So the exam content should match the course objectives. They also suggest that medical schools use a range of assessment techniques for testing the curricular outcomes. This is important as different assessment techniques measure different competence levels.

Formative and Summative Assessment

Assessments may either be formative or summative. Formative assessment promotes the development of the resident, which is usually through feedback on their performance. Formative assessments in medical education are usually used as a tool for identifying the students' strengths and weaknesses, which are then used for remediation. Summative assessment provides a summary of the student's performance which can then be used to make decisions such as grades, promotion or remediation.

The term assessment for learning may be considered an alternative name for formative assessment, and again meaning assessment that is used specifically to enhance the learning process or performances, rather than just measure them

(Hargreaves, 2007). Therefore when different assessment methods are discussed below the validity of the tool, as an assessment for learning will depend on how much the tool was used and intended and lead to further learning. The difficulty with that is on occasions the extent of further learning from the assessment may be difficult to judge or calculate making the validity of the assessment challenging to dictate.

Assessment of learning is the more traditional idea of assessment where students are tested to see if they have achieved what has been intended for them. This is formally known also as summative assessment or end of program assessment. In the literature there are many instruments or tools that have been described that can be used for this type of assessment. In this assignment the most commonly used tools for summative assessment will be discussed and critiqued in brief.

Assessment Methods

More recent trends in medical education show a change in emphasis from knowledge and recall to problem solving, communication skills, attitude, professionalism and transferable skills. Therefore newer assessment methods such as portfolios have been developed and a variety of assessment tools need to be used.

Miller (1990) described a learning pyramid, which starts with the learner's cognition and moves towards a focus on the learner's behavior. Van Der Vleuten (2002) later linked a hierarchy of assessment approaches with Millers Pyramid. This model is helpful as it shows different assessment instruments at each level of the pyramid

The figure below shows Millers pyramid with each of the four levels matched with assessment approaches.

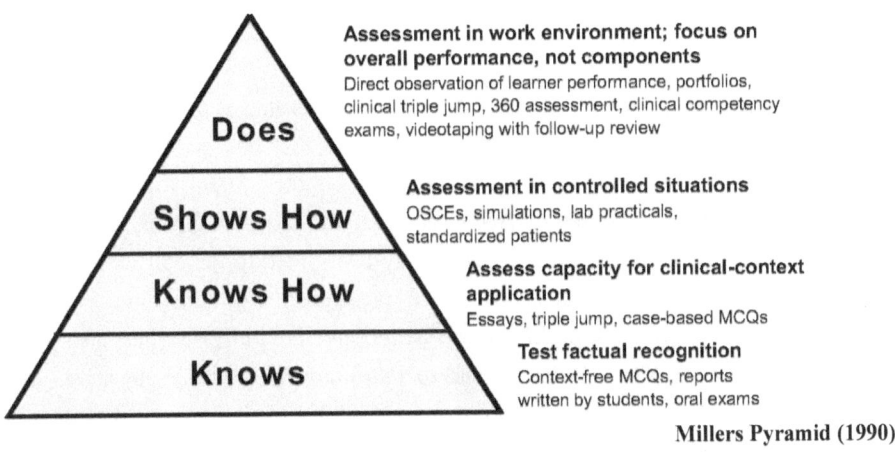

Millers Pyramid (1990)

Educators are aware of the importance of applying certain teaching methods for different curricular material. For example teaching students communication skills from reading a book would not be as ideal as from group discussion and role-plays. Similarly educators need to align teaching methods to assessment tool. In choosing an assessment tool educators need to consider the content, method and context. The content can be mapped from a blue print, which will be discussed later in more detail. The assessment method should align with the nature of the knowledge, skill or attitude to be assessed. It should be based on what provides best evidence of achievement rather than what is easiest to measure.

To select the appropriate assessment, educators should have some understanding of the strengths and weaknesses of different assessment tools. Important concepts that need to be considered are validity, reliability, and practicality.

The validity of an assessment tool is the degree to which it measures what it is supposed to measure and whether the score fails to measure the learning outcomes intended. The reliability of a test is the consistency or reproducibility of that test.

The practicality of an assessment method is also important. This usually depends on the resources that are available including cost. The cost of an assessment needs to be considered keeping in mind its benefits to teaching and learning. Van der Vleuten (1996) argued that an investment in a good assessment is also an investment in teaching and learning.

Blueprinting

As assessment needs to be valid, meaning that students that achieve the minimum performance actually have acquired the competence that has been set out in the learning objectives. An assessment blueprint facilitates the content validity of a test. The blueprint first tabulates the curricular content, and then priority is given to the more important content. The blueprint is usually distributed to the educators so they can plan the learning experience so that it is aligned with the objectives and assessment of the curriculum. In some institutions the blueprint has also been distributed to the students. The aim was to reinforce the learning objectives and deliver the intended curriculum (Coderre, et al., 2009). This can also be seen as methods of using assessment for learning. Although according to McLaughlin (2005) blueprint publication did not improve student performance but significantly increased perception of fairness of the evaluation process.

Objective Structured Clinical Examination

The OSCE is done outside the real clinical environment but is a simulation of the real environment and assesses clinical competence at the "shows how" level of millers pyramid. Students rotate through a series of structured cases where at each station specific tasks have to be performed. These skills usually involve history taking, physical examination, practical skills and counseling. These stations may include standardized patients, real patients or simulation. The marking system at each station is structured and set in advance usually in the form of a checklist.

The OSCE assesses performance and tests what students 'can do' rather than what the students know. The station or clinical encounter has three variables, which are the student, the patient, and the examiner. To be able to assess a student accurately in the same OSCE, the patient and the examiner need to be held constant across all of the different students that have to be assessed.

The OSCE has many advantages; it is practical, reliable and valid in assessing clinical competence. In general, the larger the number of stations in the OSCE, the greater the reliability and validity are. The ACGME specifies that for a minimum reliability, the OSCE needs to consist of at least 20 stations.

Another study done by Probert (2003) found that student performance in a traditional clinical final examination was not as good an indicator of rating as a junior doctor by a consultant as there was a positive relationship between student performance in a final year of OSCE and their rating as a junior doctor. Another advantage of an OSCE is that by using simulation for assessment, procedures which would usually be difficult to assess on real patients due to putting the patient at risk would now be feasible.

OSCEs may be used for formative as well as summative assessment. Feedback can be given to the student instantly so that they can respond to that information and correct the behavior. This provides a very powerful opportunity for learning and is an example of assessment for learning.

A potential disadvantage of an OSCE is that the student may prepare for the examination by memorizing the checklists or steps without fully understanding the skills in different contexts.

OSCEs can be very difficult to organize. The need detailed planning participation of many assessors, real patients, simulated patients, and administrative and technical staff. An OSCE may require an extensive budget as well as commitment from all the participants, which may be very challenging. Security may also be an issue, the more people involved in the exam the more risk in the integrity of the examination.

Traditionally MCQ testing was used for summative assessment, although it can also be used as a more formative assessment and therefore become an assessment for learning. In this case, results should be discussed with the student, areas of weakness should be highlighted and perhaps even a study plan noted.

Multiple Choice Questions

Multiple choice questions are the most commonly used assessment tool in medical education. The two most commonly used types are the A type which consists of a question followed by four or five options the second is the R type also known as extended matching. Multiple choice questions are known to test students recall or application of factual information, they therefore assess at the "knows" level of Millers pyramid. More recently multiple choice questions have been modified to include a clinical scenario, which allowed the assessment of the students application of knowledge, this format assesses at the "knows how" level of Millers pyramid.

Multiple choice questions have many advantages, which explains its frequent use in both low and high stake assessment. Their biggest advantage is the ease of delivery in that they can be delivered using computers, which later facilitates scoring. They can be delivered at multiple sites with little administrative cost. If the sample is selected well from a blueprint it can be both a reliable and valid assessment. These can then be proved by psychometrics calculating discrimination and difficulty indices.

Despite having many advantages, multiple choice questions also have a number of disadvantages including the fact that they assess knowledge of a subject rather than a deeper understanding. This can lead to a "cueing effect" where the student can recognize the correct answer from the list rather than knowing the information. Another disadvantage is that the multiple choice question does not mimic the real practice of medicine as in real life the patient does not come with a list of possible diagnoses.

Writing multiple choice questions may be costly as it is time consuming if done properly. There are many rules in multiple choice question writing to eliminate student test wiseness and irrelevant difficulty. Although this can be compensated by sharing item banks with different institutions.

Portfolios for Assessment

A Portfolio is a collection of work made by a student to document their achievements as well as their reflections. Snadden (1999) defined portfolio based learning as "the collection of evidence that learning has taken place, usually set within some agreed objectives or a negotiated set of learning activities"

The portfolio contains material that is collected by the student during their time of study where they include a critical review of the material they have learned. Portfolios can include critical incidents, reflective diary, learning plans, clinical experiences, procedure logs, operative logs, exam preparation materials, research, audits, projects, feedback reports, and improvement plans. Portfolios can be used for both formative and summative assessment.

In the assessment of portfolios the student's demonstration of learning outcome achievement is assessed. The benefit of using portfolios in assessment is that they assess at the "does" level of Millers pyramid, therefore implying competence. Portfolios may be also used for learning as it encourages reflection. Research has shown that reflection increases the degree to which students transfer what they have learned to new settings (Brasford et al., 2000). Through reflection students become more involved in their own education and engage in self-assessing and setting their own goals that is the basis of life-long learning.

Research also shows that for the use of portfolios to be successful, the role of a mentor is crucial (Finlay et al., 1998). This may be an obstacle to portfolio's success as an assessment tool as this will require a new perspective on education from both the student and the mentor and will require a significant investment of time and energy by both. This is where the role of the academic leaders is crucial for the success of this curricular change. Teachers and students will look to the leaders for support and commitment and this is where leaders can reflect this commitment by allocating sufficient funds, resources and time to allow the changes to be implemented.

Portfolio assessment has its own associated costs especially in developing the electronic portfolios but these investments can later be justified by the significant insight that is gained into the students' abilities and competence.

Peer Assessment

Peer assessment is also known as 360-degree evaluation; it was originally used in the business world then applied in medical education. This assessment tool involves many individuals evaluating the student, this includes faculty, nurses, peers, clerical workers and managers. This feedback is collected in a timely manner and shared with the student in an aggregate and anonymous fashion. The advantage of this approach to assessment is that it involves many evaluators, which helps to increase both validity and reliability. Also eventually the students skills and accuracy in self-assessment will improve with the comparison with the outside assessments. Another advantage is that peers are better at observing each other in clinical practice and therefore can sometimes give more accurate evaluations than faculty in certain circumstances.

Peer assessment is better and more commonly used in the assessment of attitudes, professionalism and communication skills therefore can be labeled as an assessment for learning. A weakness of this form of assessment is that it requires multiple evaluators, which will need managing and data collecting, which may be time consuming and challenging. Another challenge would be to train the raters so the results can be considered reliable and accurate.

Institutions also need to be aware that if peer assessment is conducted poorly, it can cause suspicion, distrust, and rivalry between the students. Despite theses weaknesses, peer assessment is becoming more popular and being used more in medical institutions as studies have shown that peer evaluations correlate highly with faculty evaluations of the rating of the same behaviors and skills (Gray, 1996).

Feedback

Although most of the assessment tools discussed above have been used primarily in assessment of learning, with minor modifications the same tools can be used as an assessment for learning. Feedback is the essential so called ingredient for "assessment for learning", therefore with any assessment tool, if feedback is given following the rules of feedback the assessment can be converted from assessment of learning to assessment for learning. Therefore the next fitting and crucial item that needs to be discussed is feedback.

Ende (1983) whose work on feedback has been crucial and still being implemented today suggested that there needs to be specific conditions to make feedback more conducive to learning. These conditions include setting an appropriate time and place, providing feedback regarding specific behaviors instead of general performance, giving feedback on decisions and actions rather than interpretations of actions, giving feedback in small digestible quantities and using a language that is non evaluative and non judgmental. Holmboe (2004) later added that an action plan critically needs to be formulated at the end of the feedback session to make it successful and allowing the learning loop to be closed.

The challenges in providing feedback based on the literature include poor participation of faculty in providing feedback as well as the quality of the feedback given. Some strategies to overcome these challenges include providing faculty development workshops to train the faculty in the importance of feedback and the best delivery methods. Another strategy would be to select a core group of faculty and train them in providing feedback. In improving the quality of feedback, the most common deficiency is the formulation of action plans. As discussed the action plan is vital in closing the learning loop and therefore needs to be emphasized.

Conclusion

Assessment drives learning and therefore the best tools and methods are the "assessments for learning". Assessment for learning improves the students motivation which engages them in their own education and setting of their own goals which make the basis of life-long learning. Assessment for learning involves commitment from the student and teacher, which transforms and enriches their relationship, and enhances the teacher's professional practice.

As in any move towards change, the role of the leaders is crucial. Leaders need to understand the features of assessment for learning as well as its differences from assessment of learning. Leaders need to involve all stakeholders addressing the concerns and facilitating the implementation. Expertise needs to be recognized in colleagues and supported while resources are provided.

References

ACGME (2003) Accreditation Council for Graduate Medical Education [website: http://www.acgme.org].

Accreditation Council for Graduate Medical Education [ACGME]. (2001– present). Outcome project. Chicago (IL): ACGME. Available from: www.acgme.org/Outcome (Accessed 7 June 2010).

Allen, B., Crosky, A., McAlpine, I., Hoffman, M., Munroe, P., (2006): A blended approach to collaborative learning: Can it make large group teaching more student-centred? 23rd annual ascilite conference.

Anita Walsh (2007): An exploration of Biggs' constructive alignment in the context of work-based learning, Assessment & Evaluation in Higher Education, 32:1, 79-87

Brown G., Manogue M., AMEE Medical Education Guide No. 22: (2001) Refreshing lecturing: a guide for lecturers. Medical Teacher 23: 231-244. 326:543-545.

Bligh, J., Prideaux, D., & Parsell, G. (2001). PRISMS: new educational strategies for medical education. Medical Education, 35(6), 520-521.

Bradley, P., Mattick K., (2008) Integration of basic and clinical sciences, Peninsula College of Medicine and Dentistry, UK - AMEE

Bransford. J., Browne, A.L., Cocking, R.R., (2000). How people learn: Brain, mind, experience, and school. (Washington DC, National Academy Press)

Clouder, L., Sellars, J., (2004). Journal of Advanced Nursing 46(3), 262–269 Reflective practice and clinical supervision: an interprofessional perspective Background.

Codderre, S., Woloscheuk, W., McLaughlin, K., (2009) Twelve tips for blueprinting, Medical teacher, Vol 31, pp 322–324.

Cutcliffe, J.R., Butterworth, T., Proctor, B., (2001). Fundamental themes in clinical supervision. London: Routledge.

Draper, S.W., Brown, M.I., (2004): Increasing interactivity in lectures using an electronic voting system, Journal of Computer Assisted Learning 20, pp81–94.

Dziuban, C.D., Hartman, J.S., Moskal, P.D., (2004). Blended Learning: Center for Applied Research, Research Bulletin, Mar: Vol 2004, No 7.

EndeJ., (1983). Feedback in clinical medical education. JAMA. ;250:777–81.

Finlay, I.G., Maughan., T.S., Webster, D.J., (1998). A randomized controlled study of portfolio learning in undergraduate cancer education. Medical Education, 32: 172-176.

Flynn, W., Vredevoogd. J., (2010)., 12 Views on Emerging Trends in Higher Education The future of learning, The Future of Learning, 4-10.

Freeth, D., Reeves, S. (2004). Learning to work together: Using presage, process and product (3P) to highlight decisions and possibilities. Journal of Interprofessional Care, 18, 43–56.

General Medical Council (1993) Tomorrow's Doctors: Recommendations on Undergraduate Medical Education (London, GMC).

General Medical Council (2002) Recommendations on Undergraduate Medical Education (London, GMC).

Gil, D. H., Heins, M., Jones, P. B., (1984). Perceptions of medical school faculty members and students on clinical clerkship feedback. Journal of Medical Education, 59, 856-864.

Glennys, P., Bligh, J., (1998). Techniques in medical education: Interprofessional learning. Postgraduate Medical Journal ; 74: 89-95

Gray, J., (1996) Global rating scales in residency education, Academic Medicine 71, pp. S55–63.

Hamdy, H., (2008) The fuzzy world of problem-based learning: Medical Teacher 30: 739-741.

Hamdy, H., Anderson, M.B., (2006) The Arabian Gulf University College of Medicine and Medical Sciences: A Successful Model of a Multinational Medical School. International Medical Education 81(12): 1085- 1090.

Hargreaves, E., (2007): The validity of collaborative assessment for learning, Assessment in Education: Principles, Policy & Practice, 14:2, 185-199

Harden, R.M., Crosby, J.R. & Davis, M.H. (1999) An introduction to outcome-based education: AMEE Guide No 14, part 1, Medical Teacher, 21(1), pp. 7–14.

Harden, R.M., (1999). AMEE Guide no 14: Outcome-based education. Part 1 – An introduction to outcome-based education. Med Teach 21(1):7–14.

Harden, R.M., Davis, M.H. & Crosby, J.R. (1997) The new Dundee medical curriculum: a whole that is greater than the sum of the parts, Medical Education, 31, pp. 264–271.

Harden, R. M., Snowden, S., & Dunn, W. R. (1984). Some educational strategies in curriculum development: the SPICES model. Medical Education, 18, 284-297.

Harden, R.M., (2002). Learning outcomes and instructional objectives: is there a difference? Medical Teacher, Vol. 24, No. 2, 151–155

Harden, R.M., (2007). Outcome-based education – the ostrich, the peacock and the beaver Medical Teacher, Vol. 29, 666–671

Harlen, W., James, M., (1997): Assessment and Learning: differences and relationships between formative and summative assessment, Assessment in Education: Principles, Policy & Practice, 4:3, 365-379

Harris P, Connolly J.F., Feeney L., (2009). Blended Learning: overview and recommendations for successful implementation. Industrial and Commercial Training;41(3):155-163.

Heinze, A., Blended Learning: An Interpretive action research study. PhD Salford Business School University of Salford, Salford, UK.

Heinze, A., Procter C., (2004). Reflections on the Use of Blended Learning. Education in a Changing Environment conference proceedings, University of Salford, Salford, Education Development Unit.

Held, S., McKimm J., (2009) Improve your lecturing: British Journal of Hospital Medicine, August, Vol 70, No 8.

Hesketh, E. A., Laidlaw. J.M., (2002). Developing the teaching instinct medical Teacher, Vol. 24, No 4, pp. 364–367

Higher Education in Europe (2009). Developments in the Bologna Process Education, Audiovisual & Culture Executive Agency

Holmboe, E.S.,Hawkins,R.E., Hutot, S.J., (2004). Direct observation of competence training: a randomized controlled trial. Annals of internal medicine, 140, pp. 874-81.

Hore,C.T., Lancashire, W., Fassett, R.G., (2009). Clinical supervision by consultants in teaching hospitals MJA; 191: 220–222

Jasper, M., (2003). Beginning Reflective Practice – Foundations in Nursing and Health Care Nelson Thornes. Cheltenham

Ker, J. (2001). Integrated learning. In J. A. Dent & R. M. Harden (Eds.), A Practical Guide for Medical Teachers (pp. 168-179). London: Churchill Livingstone.

Katherine, B., Luci, E., Zeryab, S., Alison, S., Turrock, A., Jean, K., (2011) Performance in assessment: Consensus statement and recommendations from the Ottawa conference Medical teacher vol 33:, pp370–383

Kilminster S.M., Jolly,B., Van der Vleuten C., (2002). A framework for training effective supervisors. Med Teach 24:385–389.

Kilminster, S.M., Cotterall, D., Grant, J., Jolly, B.C. (2007) AMEE Guide No. 27: Effective educational and clinical supervision. Medical Teacher, 29: 2–19.

Kilminster, S.M., Jolly, B.C., (2000). Effective supervision in clinical practice settings: a literature review. Med Educ; 34: 827–840.

McKimm, J., (2009) Curriculum and course design British Journal of Hospital Medicine, Dec: Vol 70, No 12

McLaughlin K, Lemaire J, Coderre S. (2005)a. Creating a reliable and valid blueprint for the internal medicine clerkship evaluation. Med Teach 27:544–547.

Miller, G.E., (1990) The assessment of clinical skills/competence/ performance, Academic Medicine, 65(Suppl.), pp. S63–S67.

Neher, J.O., Gordon, K.C., Meyer, B., Stevens. N., (1992). A five-step "microskills" model of clinical teaching. J Am Board Fam Pract ; 5:419-24.

Neher, J.O., Nancy, G., Stevens, M.D., (2003). The One-minute Preceptor: Shaping the Teaching Conversation Family Medicine Fam Med;35(6):391-3.

Norcini J, Burch V. 2007. Workplace-based assessment as an educational tool: AMEE Guide No.31. Med Teach 41(10):926–934.

NSW Institute of Medical Education and Training. Trainee in difficulty. A handbook for Directors of Prevocational Education and Training. Sydney: NSW IMET, 2009.

Perkins, D., (1993) Teaching for understanding. American Educator: The Professional Journal of the American Federation of Teachers 17(3): 8,28-35.

Prideaux, D., (2000). The emperor's new clothes: from objectives to outcomes, Medical Education, 34, pp. 168–169.

Prideaux, D., (2003) ABC of learning and teaching in Medicine: Curriculum, BMJ 2003: 326: 268-270.

Probert, C.S., Cahil, D.J., Mccann, G.L., Ben-S, Y., (2003) Traditional finals and OSCEs in predicting consultant and self-reported clinical skills of PRHOs: a pilot study, Medical Education, 37, pp. 597–602.

Reed D.A., Wright, S.M., (2010). Role Models in Medicine. In: Mentoring in Academic Medicine, Humphrey H. APC Press, Philadelphia, PA, pp. 67-81

Sloan, G.,(2005). Clinical supervision: beginning the supervisory relationship British Journal of Nursing, Vol 14, No 17

Sloan, G., (2006). Clinical Supervision in Mental Health Nursing. Whurr Plublishers Ltd, England.

Snadden, D., (1999) AMEE Education Guide No. 11 (revised): Portfolio- based learning and assessment in medical education, Medical Teacher, 4, pp. 370–386.

Standards for Licensure and Accreditation (2011). Commission for Academic Accreditation Ministry of Higher Education and Scientific Research United Arab Emirates

Steinert, Y., Snell, L.S., (1999) Interactive lecturing: strategies for increasing participation in large group presentations. Medical Teacher 21: 37-42.

Swaffield, S., (2011): Getting to the heart of authentic Assessment for Learning, Assessment in Education: Principles, Policy & Practice, 18:4, 433-449

The Universities and the National Framework of Qualifications (2005). Irish Universities Association

UAE Qualification Framework (2011). Working Draft Version A003, UAE National Qualifications Authority

Vardi, I., (2012): Effectively feeding forward from one written assessment task to the next, Assessment & Evaluation in Higher Education, DOI:10.1080/02602938.2012.670197

Van Der Vleuten, C.P.M., (1996) The assessment of professional competence: developments, research and practical implications, Advances in Health Sciences Education, 1(1), pp. 41–67.

William T., Branch, Jr., Paranjape, A., (2002). Feedback and Reflection: Teaching Methods for Clinical Settings Acad. Med. ;77:1185–1188.

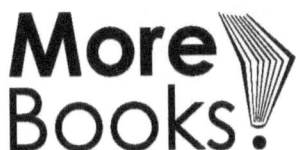
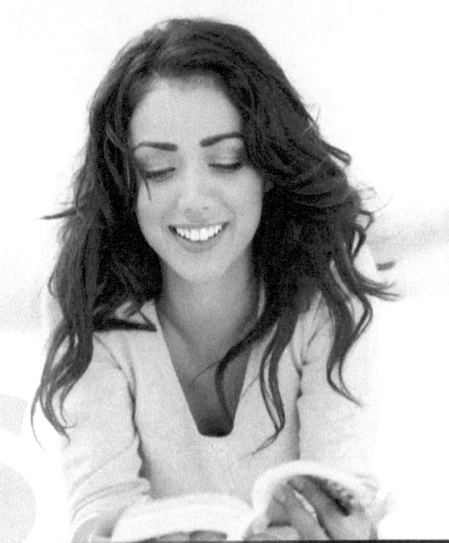

I want morebooks!

Buy your books fast and straightforward online - at one of the world's fastest growing online book stores! Environmentally sound due to Print-on-Demand technologies.

Buy your books online at
www.get-morebooks.com

Kaufen Sie Ihre Bücher schnell und unkompliziert online – auf einer der am schnellsten wachsenden Buchhandelsplattformen weltweit!
Dank Print-On-Demand umwelt- und ressourcenschonend produziert.

Bücher schneller online kaufen
www.morebooks.de

OmniScriptum Marketing DEU GmbH
Heinrich-Böcking-Str. 6-8
D - 66121 Saarbrücken
Telefax: +49 681 93 81 567-9

info@omniscriptum.com
www.omniscriptum.com

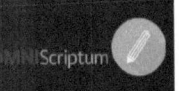

www.ingramcontent.com/pod-product-compliance
Lightning Source LLC
Chambersburg PA
CBHW031547210526
45464CB00003B/1185